YOUR KNOWLEDGE HAS VALUE

AF138323

- We will publish your bachelor's and master's thesis, essays and papers

- Your own eBook and book - sold worldwide in all relevant shops

- Earn money with each sale

Upload your text at www.GRIN.com and publish for free

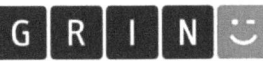

Applicability of the Braden Skala for Pressure Ulcer Prevention in the Intensive Care Unit

Stefanel Bulea

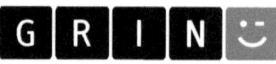

Bibliographic information published by the German National Library:

The German National Library lists this publication in the National Bibliography; detailed bibliographic data are available on the Internet at http://dnb.dnb.de.

ISBN: 9783389085455
This book is also available as an ebook.

© GRIN Publishing GmbH
Trappentreustraße 1
80339 München

All rights reserved

Print and binding: Books on Demand GmbH, Norderstedt, Germany
Printed on acid-free paper from responsible sources.

The present work has been carefully prepared. Nevertheless, authors and publishers do not incur liability for the correctness of information, notes, links and advice as well as any printing errors.

GRIN web shop: https://www.grin.com/document/1513296

Stefanel Bulea

Research Paper

Applicability of the Braden Skala
For Pressure Ulcer Prevention
In the Intensive Care Unit

Analysis and Synergy with

Complementary Preventive Care Measures

I

This paper was originally published in German under the title *'Anwendbarkeit der Braden-Skala für die Dekubitusprophylaxe auf der Intensivstation'* and has been translated into English by the author.

Stefanel Bulea has been a Registered Nurse in Germany since 2021, holding a Bachelor's Degree in Nursing, obtained in Romania in 2016. This paper was written during his further training as a practical instructor in nursing (Praxisanleiter in der Pflege).

Table of Contents

List of Abbreviations

BS	Braden-Skala
DNQP	Deutsche Netzwerk für Qualitätsentwicklung
IS	Intensivstation
MOF	Multi Organ failure
CVC	Central Venous Catheter

1   Introduction

Florence Nightingale (1860) emphasized the importance of patient safety with the apt words: "The very first requirement in a hospital is that it should do the sick no harm." This fundamental principle of health ethics underscores the obligation of hospitals to prioritize the well-being of patients above all else.

Today, this maxim is particularly relevant, especially in intensive care units (ICU), where nurses, doctors, and other medical professionals face complex and diverse challenges daily. Time is extremely precious in these units, as every second slips away in the pursuit of quick decisions.

In this environment, every detail is crucial, and no sound can be ignored. An abnormal heart rate immediately triggers the monitors' alarms, demanding attention. An oxygen saturation below the threshold activates the ventilator's alarm. Yet there is also a silent enemy that develops insidiously - pressure ulcers (decubitus).

These skin lesions are caused by prolonged pressure on certain body areas, which impairs local blood circulation (ischemia), leading to tissue damage (Daumann, 2018, p. 45). The risk of developing pressure ulcers is further influenced by the patient's critical condition, including sedation, prolonged immobility, and severe comorbidities (Daumann, 2018, p. 46).

Like a "parasite," pressure ulcers exploit the patient's weakness and can cause significant damage if not properly treated. Therefore, the treatment, and especially the prevention, of pressure ulcers is an essential component of intensive care and represents a challenge for medical staff, who must remain constantly vigilant.

One of the most important contributions in this area was made by Barbara Braden and Nancy Bergstrom. In 1980, they developed a scale for assessing the risk of pressure ulcers. This scale aims to systematically evaluate six risk factors: the patient's sensory perception, the skin's exposure to moisture, the patient's activity level, the ability to change body position, nutritional status, and the extent of friction and shear to which the patient's skin is exposed (Bergstrom, Braden, Laguzza & Holman, 1987).

However, applying the Braden Scale (BS) in the ICU is particularly challenging, as patients are often immobilized, receive parenteral nutrition, and are under sedative medications, which can significantly impair sensory perception and mobility. These specific conditions increase the risk of pressure ulcers, which in turn raises questions about the validity of the BS in certain aspects (Hyun et al., 2013).

Therefore, an accurate and regular reassessment of the BS's adaptability in such situations is necessary. This paper aims to analyze the extent to which the BS is applicable in the ICU for the prevention of pressure ulcers and to identify potential synergies with complementary preventive care measures.

First, the characteristic features of ICU patients, as well as their specific medical and nursing needs, will be described in detail. Then, the BS as an assessment tool will be examined, with a critical evaluation of the relevance of its six criteria in the context of intensive care. Finally, additional measures for the prevention of pressure ulcers will be presented, and their potential synergies with the BS will be discussed.

This investigation aims to derive practical recommendations to optimize pressure ulcer prevention in the ICU, improve care quality, and enhance patient well-being. It seeks to provide both theoretical and practical insights for medical nursing practice and to sustainably reduce the incidence of pressure ulcers.

2 ICU Patient Characteristics

2.1 General Description of the ICU Patient Population

The ICU patient population has specific demographic and health characteristics that increase the risk of developing pressure ulcers. ICU patients are often older and tend to suffer from chronic conditions such as diabetes, heart failure, and kidney failure. These conditions worsen overall health and heighten vulnerability to pressure ulcers. According to the DecubISs study (2021), the prevalence of pressure ulcers in ICUs is 27%, with 59% of these injuries attributed to the ICU stay (Labeau et al., 2021).

According to the National Pressure Ulcer Advisory Panel, patients suffering from severe and often life-threatening conditions such as sepsis, multi-organ failure (MOF), or severe trauma require intensive medical interventions, which significantly increase the risk of pressure ulcers (Haesler, NPUAP, 2014).

2.2 Specific Medical and Nursing Care Needs

Next, we will examine to what extent the specific medical and nursing needs influence the development of pressure ulcers in ICU patients, with a focus on the need for catecholamines, sedation, and nutrition.

2.2.1 Relationship between Catecholamine and Risk of Pressure Ulcers

Catecholamines are endogenous hormones produced in the adrenal medulla. The most important ones are adrenaline, noradrenaline, and dopamine. These hormones play a crucial role in regulating heart rate, blood pressure, and blood sugar levels (Everts & Heiling, 2021, p. 188).

There are also synthetic drugs classified as catecholamines, known under various trade names, such as Suprarenin (adrenaline), Arterenol (noradrenaline), and Dobutrex (dopamine) (Kany & Meixner, 2018, p. 38).

In the ICU, catecholamines like adrenaline and noradrenaline are often used to stabilize blood pressure in critically ill patients.

The increased need for catecholamines can raise the risk of pressure ulcers, as these substances cause vasoconstriction, which reduces blood flow to the skin and underlying tissues. Reduced tissue perfusion leads to inadequate oxygen and nutrient supply, promoting the development of pressure ulcers (De Backer, Critical Care, 2023).

2.2.2 Effects of Sedation on Patient Mobility

Deep sedation is required in cases of severe neurological conditions, after resuscitation during the cooling phase, and for surgical necessities such as polytrauma and increased intracranial pressure. It is also used for managing elevated intracranial pressure and to suppress rapid spontaneous breathing in severe acute respiratory distress syndrome (Everts & Heiling, 2021, p. 65). Important medications for sedation include propofol, Ketanest, and midazolam (Everts & Heiling, 2021, p. 66).

Sedated patients are significantly restricted in their ability to move, which increases the risk of pressure ulcers. The limited movement prevents patients from independently changing their position, leading to prolonged pressure on certain areas of the body. Additionally, sedation impairs sensory perception, making it difficult for patients to feel pressure points and respond accordingly (Hyun et al., 2013).

2.2.3 Nutritional Needs and Pressure Ulcer Risk in Tube Feeding

Adequate nutrition is crucial for skin health and the prevention of pressure ulcers. In ICU patients, artificial nutrition presents a particular challenge. Parenteral nutrition can lead to insufficient intake of essential nutrients necessary for skin integrity and wound healing. Malnutrition and specific nutrient deficiencies, such as a lack of protein, increase the risk of pressure ulcers by weakening the skin and underlying tissues (Blumenstein et al., 2014; Sauer et al., 2019).

Enteral nutrition is often provided through tube feeding, administered via percutaneous endoscopic gastrostomy (PEG), percutaneous endoscopic jejunostomy (PEJ), or nasogastric tubes. However, these methods can cause pressure points and local inflammation, requiring additional care and monitoring (Kalde, Vogt, & Kolbig, 2022, pp. 100-124).

In clinical practice, there are also situations where tube feeding alone is insufficient to meet the patient's nutritional needs. In such cases, parenteral nutrition plays a critical role. A balanced mix of amino acids, glucose, lipids, electrolytes, and trace elements can be administered to meet daily nutritional requirements. Since parenteral nutrition can lead to vein irritation and other complications, it is delivered via a central venous catheter (CVC) (Everts & Heiling, 2021, p. 429).

A CVC can indirectly influence the risk of pressure ulcers, as it serves as an entry point for catecholamines and sedative medications and can also be a potential source of infection due to local tissue damage (ESPEN, 2020; Frontiers in Medicine, 2022).

Whether in hospitals, nursing homes, or home care, the use of appropriate risk assessment tools is essential. As Hippocrates emphasized in his writings around 400 B.C., "It is better to prevent than to cure," and this principle is fundamental to modern medicine. One of the most used risk assessment tools is the Braden Scale (BS), which helps assess the risk of pressure ulcers in patients. The following section will examine in detail whether the BS is also suitable for use in ICUs.

3 The Braden Scale as an Assessment Tool in the Intensive Care Unit

The Braden Scale (BS) was developed in the 1980s by Barbara Braden and Nancy Bergstrom to systematically assess the risk of pressure ulcers. Initially designed for use in various care settings, the scale aims to quantify the risk and guide the implementation of preventive measures (A. Floyd et al., 2021).

3.1. Origin and Development of the Braden Scale

The BS evaluates six different factors: sensory perception, moisture, activity, mobility, nutrition, and friction/shear. Each of these factors is rated on a scale from 1 to 4 (with friction/shear rated from 1 to 3), where lower scores indicate a higher risk. The total score ranges from 6 to 23, with lower overall scores signifying a higher risk for developing pressure ulcers (Bergstrom, Braden, Laguzza & Holman, 1987).

According to Braden (1987), the risk levels are classified as follows: low risk (more than 15 points), moderate risk (14-12 points), high risk (11-9 points), and very high risk (less than 9 points) (Bergstrom, Braden, Laguzza & Holman, 1987).

According to the healthcare standards of the Gesundheitsverbund Landkreis Konstanz GmbH (2020), it has been observed that there are additional factors influencing the assessment of pressure ulcer risk. If one or more additional factors are present, the patient is classified into the next higher risk category. These factors include noncompliance, cachexia, sedatives, hemiplegia, and paraplegia.

3.2.   Relevance of the Six Braden Scale Criteria for ICU Patients

3.2.1. Sensory Perception in Sedated ICU Patients

Deep sedation is necessary in various critical situations in the ICU, such as patients undergoing prolonged mechanical ventilation, during invasive or painful medical procedures, to control increased intracranial pressure, and to suppress rapid breathing rates in ARDS cases. However, deep sedation carries risks, including an increased risk of pressure ulcers due to prolonged immobility and reduced sensory perception (Everts & Heiling, 2021, pp. 64-65).

In the ICU, the level of sedation is carefully monitored using the Richmond Agitation-Sedation Scale (RASS). This scale allows for the assessment of a patient's agitation or sedation level on a scale from -5 (deep sedation) to +4 (agitation) to ensure that each patient is sedated appropriately based on their specific medical needs (Everts & Heiling, 2021, pp. 64-65).

Furthermore, evaluating sensory perception is crucial because the reduction of this perception due to sedation directly increases the risk of developing pressure ulcers. This highlights the need for targeted prevention strategies in sedated patients, such as regular repositioning and the use of pressure-relieving mattresses (A. Floyd et al., 2021). Sensory perception becomes even more relevant when sedation is gradually reduced to wake the patient from an induced coma.

In this phase, close monitoring and adjustments in care are necessary to continue minimizing the risk of pressure ulcers, as patients begin to feel pain and discomfort again and react accordingly (Haesler, NPUAP, 2014).

3.2.2. Moisture Assessment in Patients with Multi-Organ Failure

Multi-organ failure (MOF), particularly kidney failure, often leads to increased moisture levels due to skin exudation or incontinence. Assessing moisture is essential to minimize the risk of pressure ulcers. The BS considers moisture as one of its six main factors, making its use particularly relevant for these patients (A. Floyd et al., 2021).

Accurate fluid intake and output monitoring is crucial. This includes precise documentation of all fluids administered and those excreted, such as urine, drainage, gastric secretions, and sweat (Garcia et al., 2017).

Specific considerations are necessary for patients with particular MOF conditions. In kidney failure, strict monitoring of fluid balance and adjustments to diuretic dosing or dialysis frequency may be required. Heart failure often necessitates limiting fluid intake and using diuretics or inotropic medications to support heart function. In liver failure, assessing ascites and performing paracentesis when needed is important. These measures are crucial to minimize complications and improve the patients' quality of life (Garcia et al., 2017).

Nurses use the BS to assess skin moisture levels and implement appropriate measures to reduce moisture and protect the skin (A. Floyd et al., 2021).

Incontinence, especially urinary incontinence, is a common issue in ICU patients that can lead to skin damage and an increased risk of infection. Effective management includes regular skin inspections and cleaning, the use of incontinence aids such as pads and diapers, and protective creams to prevent skin irritation. Regular moisture assessments help ensure timely interventions, such as changing dressings, preventing moisture buildup with protective creams, or frequent repositioning to prevent skin damage. These measures are critical for minimizing complications and improving patient quality of life (Danzer & Kamphausen, 2016, pp. 141-149).

3.2.3. Activity Level and Pressure Ulcer Risk in Intubated Patients

Intubated patients are often immobilized, significantly increasing their risk of developing pressure ulcers. Although the activity level in these patients is obviously low, assessing this factor with the BS remains relevant for comprehensively understanding and managing the overall risk of pressure ulcers (A. Floyd et al., 2021).

Even though the low activity level in intubated patients is evident, formal assessment helps document the severity of immobility and serves as a basis for nursing interventions (A. Floyd et al., 2021).

The formal documentation of low activity levels supports nurses in planning and implementing structured and consistent preventive measures, such as regular repositioning and the use of specialized pressure-relieving mattresses. These interventions are crucial to preventing pressure ulcers by reducing pressure on vulnerable body areas (Truong, A.D., 2019).

Assessing activity levels serves not only for risk evaluation but also for documentation and communication within the care team. Clear and systematic documentation supports shift handovers and continuous care planning (Truong, A.D., 2019).

3.2.4. Mobility in Patients Dependent on Repositioning Plans

As discussed in the previous section on activity, limited mobility is a significant risk factor for the development of pressure ulcers. The BS evaluates both activity level and mobility to enable a comprehensive risk assessment. These two factors are closely related and influence the overall risk of pressure ulcers (Truong, A.D., 2019).

Studies have shown that regular repositioning and mobility promotion are essential for reducing the risk of pressure ulcers. Even in patients entirely dependent on repositioning plans, the BS's mobility assessment remains relevant, as it provides an evidence-based foundation for prevention strategies (A. Floyd et al., 2021). Mobility assessment enables the creation of individualized care plans that account for the patient's specific mobility level.

This is particularly important for patients dependent on repositioning, as standard repositioning intervals and techniques must be tailored to individual mobility and health conditions (Gillespie B. et al., 2020).

3.2.5. Nutritional Adequacy in Patients on Tube Feeding

Malnutrition impairs wound healing by causing stagnation, prolonged inflammatory phases, reduced fibroblast activity, defective neo angiogenesis, unstable collagen, and increased tissue fragility. It also increases the risk of wound healing complications, such as suppuration and dehiscence, complicates infection control, and negatively affects wound closure and suture stability (Danzer & Kamphausen, 2016, pp. 135-140).

The BS evaluates nutrition as one of the six key factors for assessing pressure ulcer risk. Patients can score a maximum of 4 points (good nutrition) if they receive all necessary nutrients in adequate amounts. This also applies to patients receiving tube feeding, as tube feeding formulas are designed to provide complete nutrition (Hyun et al., 2013).

As noted in section 3.2.2, alongside ensuring adequate nutrient intake, moisture management should also be considered. A balanced diet helps strengthen the skin barrier and minimize the risk of pressure ulcers, especially when combined with effective moisture management strategies (Garcia et al., 2017).

For patients with pressure ulcers, therapeutic nutrition requires a daily intake of 1.6-2 grams of protein per kilogram of body weight and 40-50 kcal per kilogram of body weight in carbohydrates to ensure protein synthesis necessary for wound healing. However, enteral nutrition must be regularly adjusted based on the patient's tolerance of the formula. Such nutritional adjustments can cause gastrointestinal issues like diarrhea or vomiting (Danzer & Kamphausen, 2016, p. 139).

3.2.6. Consideration of Friction and Shear in ICU Patients

Friction and shear are critical factors in the development of pressure ulcers, particularly in ICU patients. Shear forces occur when skin layers or underlying tissues shift against each other, often during repositioning or moving of patients. These forces can damage blood vessels in the skin, impair circulation, and lead to skin and tissue damage, even when direct pressure on the skin is not particularly high (Gefen, 2008).

Healthcare providers should be aware of the risks of friction and shear and learn techniques to minimize these forces. Good training can improve care quality and prevent pressure ulcers (Labeau et al., 2021).

So far, the application of the BS in the ICU has been explored, although some aspects of the condition of ICU patients increase the risk of pressure ulcers. The synergy between the systematic use of the BS and targeted nursing interventions can help mitigate this risk effectively.

The following chapter will describe additional measures based on the BS that allow for a comprehensive assessment and targeted prevention of pressure ulcers.

4. Complementary Measures for pressure Ulcer Prevention in ICU

4.1. Continuous Pressure Relief and Positioning

Continuous pressure relief and proper positioning are crucial in minimizing the risk of pressure ulcers. Various positioning techniques can help evenly distribute pressure and relieve specific areas of the body. The 30-degree lateral position (left and right) reduces direct pressure on the sacrum and hips. Patients are tilted slightly to the side, redistributing pressure to other areas of the body (Danzer & Kamphausen, 2016).

Additionally, the 135-degree prone position (left and right) relieves pressure on the back and redistributes pressure to the front of the body. Patients lie at an angle on their stomachs, helping to relieve pressure from common areas such as the sacrum and heels (Danzer & Kamphausen, 2016, pp. 51-58).

Another important technique is prone positioning, which is especially used in patients with severe lung failure (e.g., ARDS). This position improves oxygenation and reduces the risk of pressure ulcers on the back. Furthermore, the V-A-T-I positioning method is used for pneumonia prevention (Danzer & Kamphausen, 2016, p. 57).

The various V-A-T-I positions promote ventilation of different lung sections and reduce the risk of pneumonia (Danzer & Kamphausen, 2016, p. 57).

Different types of mattresses also contribute to pressure relief and can minimize the risk of pressure ulcers. Foam mattresses are a common and cost-effective option that distribute body weight evenly and provide moderate pressure relief, particularly for patients at low to moderate risk of pressure ulcers. Low-pressure air mattresses, which are available with or without motors, offer greater adaptability (Danzer & Kamphausen, 2016, pp. 59-62).

Motorized variants continuously adjust the pressure, making them advantageous for patients at high risk of pressure ulcers. Non-motorized air mattresses can be manually inflated to meet the individual needs of the patient (Danzer & Kamphausen, 2016, pp. 59-62).

4.2. Skin Care and Moisture Control

Effective skin care and moisture control are essential in reducing the risk of pressure ulcers. Preventive dressings on intact skin, such as on the nose or heels, can significantly reduce the incidence of pressure ulcers. These dressings act as a protective barrier, preventing direct friction and pressure on vulnerable skin areas (Everts & Heiling, 2021, p. 73).

The use of ointments, pastes, powders, oils, as well as tanning and disinfecting solutions, is contraindicated in patients at high risk of pressure ulcers, as they can further irritate and burden the skin. Measures that promote blood circulation, such as vigorous rubbing or massages, should also be avoided, as they do not show any proven improvement in blood circulation and instead increase the risk of skin damage (Everts & Heiling, 2021, p. 73).

Skin care should always be gentle, with the skin kept dry to prevent moisture and related skin damage. It is important to use mild cleaning agents and soft towels to avoid irritating the skin. Gentle cleaning and drying of the skin without excessive pressure are key steps in maintaining skin health and preventing pressure ulcers (Danzer & Kamphausen, 2016, pp. 141-149).

4.3. Training of Nursing Staff in Pressure Ulcer Prevention

The training of nursing staff in pressure ulcer prevention is a critical aspect of care quality and patient safety in healthcare settings. A pressure ulcer, also known as a decubitus ulcer, is a localized injury to the skin and underlying tissue caused by prolonged pressure or shear forces. Prevention of these injuries requires specific knowledge and skills from nursing staff (Deutsches Netzwerk für Qualitätsentwicklung in der Pflege [DNQP], 2017).

Updating and further educating nursing staff is of great importance to stay up to date with the latest research and techniques. Regular refresher courses and continuing education are necessary to evaluate training programs and adapt them to new insights and techniques (National Pressure Ulcer Advisory Panel, 2014).

4.4. Implementation of Wound Management Protocols

The implementation of wound management protocols in the ICU, which include early mobilization of patients within the first 72 hours, is crucial. Concepts such as the Bobath and kinesthetic approaches, along with a structured stepwise mobilization plan, can significantly improve patient mobility and reduce the risk of pressure ulcers. The combination of these approaches provides a comprehensive framework for promoting mobility and supporting wound healing in critically ill patients (Everts & Heiling, 2021, p. 392).

Medical and nursing wound management offers a structured approach to wound care, including wound diagnosis, identification of causes, treatment planning, causal therapy, addressing underlying causes, as well as documentation and monitoring of progress. This method allows for effective and holistic wound treatment (Daumann, 2018, p. 79).

5. Conclusion

To evaluate the applicability of the Braden Scale (BS) for pressure ulcer prevention in the intensive care unit, this paper examined the use of the BS for pressure ulcer prophylaxis in intensive care and its synergy with complementary preventive measures. The BS takes into account six main factors: sensory perception, moisture level, physical activity, mobility, nutritional status, and friction and shear forces. Intensive care needs, such as sedation, immobility, and specific nutritional requirements, increase the risk of pressure ulcers and present particular challenges for the effective application of the scale.

The results show that the systematic use of the BS, combined with targeted prevention strategies, can effectively reduce the risk of pressure ulcers. Key complementary measures include continuous pressure relief, proper positioning, effective skin care, moisture control, and the training of nursing staff. These measures help minimize pressure on vulnerable areas of the body and promote skin health.

Continuous pressure relief through various positioning techniques and specialized mattresses, along with gentle skin care, is essential. Training nursing staff ensures that current knowledge and techniques for pressure ulcer prevention are applied. Implementing pressure ulcer and wound management protocols, including early mobilization and specialized care concepts, improves care quality and reduces the risk of pressure ulcers.

Overall, the BS remains a valuable tool for risk assessment, especially when combined with preventive measures. This systematic approach can improve care quality in the ICU and sustainably reduce the incidence of pressure ulcers, significantly enhancing patient well-being.

This translation preserves the formal and professional tone of the original text while ensuring clarity and flow in English.

References

Books

Daumann, S. (2018). Wundmanagement und Wunddokumentation, Kohlhammer. 5. Auflage

Danzer, S., & Kamphausen, U. (2016). Dekubitus Prophylaxe und Therapie Kohlhammer. 1. Auflage

Kalde, S., Vogt, M., & Kolbig, N. (2002). Enterale Ernährung München. Urban & Fischer. 3. Auflage

Kany, A., & Meixner, I. (2018). Taschenwissen Intensivpflege Elsevier, 1.Auflage

Everts, K., & Heiling, M. (2021). Intensiv- und Anästhesiepflege: 1000 Fragen 1000 Antworten. Elsevier. 1. Auflage

Nightingale, F. (2008). *Notes on Nursing: What It Is and What It Is Not, and Other Writings*. Kaplan Publishing. (Originalarbeit veröffentlicht 1860)

Journal Articles

Bulea, S. (2024). Anwendbarkeit der Braden-Skala für die Dekubitusprophylaxe auf der Intensivstation. GRIN Publishing.

Bergstrom, N., Braden, B. J., Laguzza, A., & Holman, V. (1987). The Braden Scale for Predicting Pressure Sore Risk. Nursing Research, 36(4), 205-210.

Blumenstein, I., Shastri, Y. M., & Stein, J. (2014). Gastroenteric tube feeding: Techniques, problems and solutions. World Journal of Gastroenterology, 20(26), 8505-8524. https://doi.org/10.3748/wjg.v20.i26.8505

De Backer, D., & Foulon, P. (2019). Minimizing catecholamines and optimizing perfusion. Critical Care, 23(Suppl 1), 149. https://doi.org/10.1186/s13054-019-2433-6

Ely, E. W., Shintani, A., Truman, B., Speroff, T., Gordon, S. M., Harrell, F. E., Inouye, S. K., Bernard, G. R., & Dittus, R. S. (2004). Delirium as a predictor of mortality in mechanically ventilated patients in the intensive care unit. JAMA, 291(14), 1753-1762. https://doi.org/10.1001/jama.291.14.1753

Gefen, A. (2007). The biomechanics of sitting-acquired pressure ulcers in patients with spinal cord injury or lesions. International Wound Journal, 4(3), 222-231. https://doi.org/10.1111/j.1742-481X.2007.00330.x

Hyun, S., Vermillion, B., Newton, C., Fall, M., Li, X., Kaewprag, P., Moffatt-Bruce, S., & Lenz, E. R. (2013). Predictive validity of the Braden scale for patients in intensive care units. American Journal of Critical Care, 22(6), 514-520. https://doi.org/10.4037/ajcc2013991

Labeau, S. O., Afonso, E., Benbenishty, J., Blackwood, B., Boulanger, C., Brett, S. J., ... & Blot, S. I. (2021). Prevalence, associated factors and outcomes of pressure injuries in adult intensive care unit patients: the DecubISs study. Intensive Care Medicine, 47(2), 160-169. https://doi.org/10.1007/s00134-020-06234-9

Truong, A. D., Fan, E., Brower, R. G., & et al. (2009). Bench-to-bedside review: Mobilizing patients in the intensive care unit – from pathophysiology to clinical trials. Critical Care, 13, 216. https://doi.org/10.1186/cc7885

Internet Sources/ Websites

ESPEN. (2020). ESPEN guidelines on clinical nutrition. https://www.espen.org/files/ESPEN-Guidelines/ESPEN_practical_and_partially_revised_guideline_Clinical_nutrition_in_t he_intensive_care_unit.pdf

National Pressure Ulcer Advisory Panel, European Pressure Ulcer Advisory Panel and Pan Pacific Pressure Injury Alliance. (2014). Prevention and Treatment of Pressure Ulcers: Clinical Practice Guideline. Emily Haesler (Ed.). Cambridge Media:

Osborne Park, Western Australia.
https://cdn.ymaws.com/npiap.com/resource/resmgr/2014_guideline.pdf

Floyd, N. A., Dominguez-Cancino, K. A., Butler, L. G., Rivera-Lozada, O., Leyva-Moral, J. M., & Palmieri, P. A. (n.d.). The effectiveness of care bundles including the Braden Scale for preventing hospital acquired pressure ulcers in older adults hospitalized in ISs: A systematic review. Journal Name. Advance online publication.
https://opennursingjournal.com/VOLUME/15/PAGE/74/FULLTEXT/

Garcia, M., Thomas, L., & Martinez, A. (2017). Fluid intake and output in IS patients. Critical Care Nursing Quarterly, 113-161.
https://www.baccn.org/static/uploads/resources/WFCCN_e_book_SG_edits_Oct_29_17_97Q3V6x.pdf

Gillespie, B. M., Walker, R. M., Latimer, S. L., Thalib, L., Whitty, J. A., McInnes, E., & Chaboyer, W. P. (2020). Repositioning for pressure injury prevention in adults. Cochrane Database of Systematic Reviews.
https://www.cochranelibrary.com/cdsr/doi/10.1002/14651858.CD009958.pub3/full

Guidelines (Standard Working Procedures)

Deutsches Netzwerk für Qualitätsentwicklung in der Pflege (Hrsg.). (2017). Expertenstandard Dekubitusprophylaxe in der Pflege: 2. Aktualisierung 2017 einschließlich Kommentierung und Literaturstudie.

Gesundheitsverbund Landkreis Konstanz GmbH. (2020). Pflege-Assesment-Skalen (Risikoenschätzungs-Skalen). Gesundheitsministerium Baden-Württemberg.

YOUR KNOWLEDGE HAS VALUE

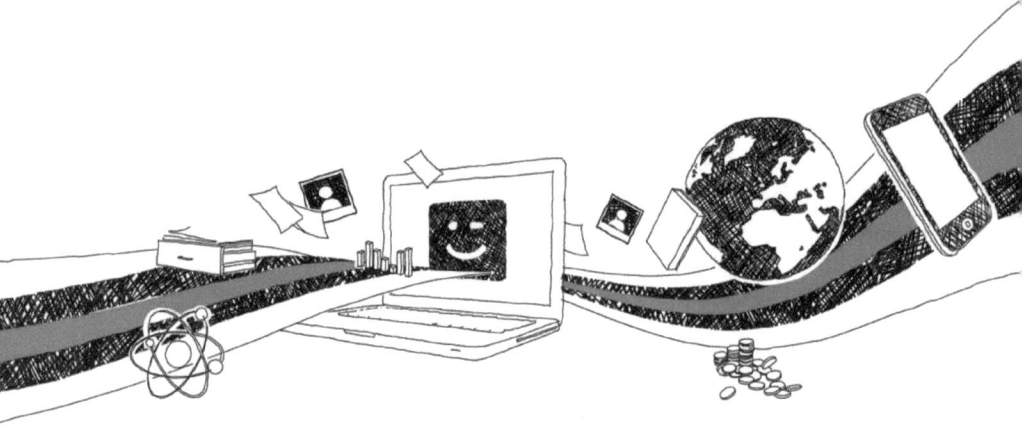

- We will publish your bachelor's and
  master's thesis, essays and papers

- Your own eBook and book -
  sold worldwide in all relevant shops

- Earn money with each sale

Upload your text at www.GRIN.com
and publish for free

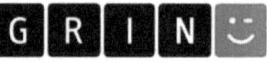